Infused Water

"Complete guide on healthy herbs and their benefits. Recipes of infusions and herbal teas to detox, relief stress, drain, lose weight, digest, regain energy and vitality"

Charles Thompson

Contents

Infused Water

Introduction

Winter is a season in its beautiful way, full of suggestive atmospheres, a unique light, a harsh climate, but which evokes a desire for warmth, comforting intimacy, which inevitably brings us back to our childhood when winter meant snowball and hot chocolate battles. Unfortunately, we are no longer children, and certain aspects of this season have become more of a nuisance than a pleasure. The low temperatures and humidity that characterize it put a strain on our body and our health. The immune system is constantly under attack, heating in homes and shops makes it all too easy to get cold when you go out, and, in general, the energy languishes, making us feel the urgent desire to hibernate and wake up in the spring. This state of affairs often conditions even the mood. Winter is characterized by fewer hours of light, bad weather, and cold: there is no need to be meteoropathic to suffer from mood swings, anxiety, lethargy, anxiety, lethargy. It is a normal consequence of the climate, but, sometimes, this seasonal depression makes it difficult to concentrate on studying, working, and serenely facing everyday life. There are many ways to overcome the winter season without losing a smile and, above all, health. It is necessary to adopt a few simple rules of life, such as avoiding keeping the heating too high, so as not to run into cold strokes when going out, make sure that there is the right humidity in the house, so as not to stress the mucous membranes too much and help respiratory tract, maintaining regular schedules, feeding properly and not giving up going out, to fight depression and to keep away sadness and tiredness. But there are other, absolutely natural aids that can help us avoid the ailments that

affect the body and spirit in winter, and fight them. We
are talking about herbal teas and infusions, special and
irreplaceable friends, 'grandmother' remedies, but always
effective, against colds, flu, coughs, and insomnia,
sadness, and anxiety. Not to mention that Christmas
offers us innumerable occasions to taste herbs and spices
as fragrant and exquisite ingredients to enrich our dishes
of the Festival! Who can resist the unmistakable aroma of
cinnamon, cloves, ginger, not only as a flu remedy but
also only as comfort on colder days? These drinks can
help us strengthen our immune system and keep seasonal
ailments away. In addition, in this guide, you will also find
recipes of cold infusions to taste during the summer.
Therefore, let's discover the difference between infusions
and herbal teas, preparations, recipes, trying to learn how
they can be useful for our well-being.

Chapter 1: Herbal Teas

Preparing a herbal tea or is a moment of relaxation that we should give ourselves more often. It can be said that there is a right herbal tea recipe for every occasion, just knowing how to choose it according to your needs but also your tastes. The herbal teas can be made with one or more herbs or plants depending on the effect you want to achieve; they also calibrate the flavor by adding, for example, red fruits, anise, mint, or something else that serves to make the mix more pleasant. There are herbal tea recipes for those who want to have natural help to lose weight, detoxify the body, facilitate digestion, regain their intestinal regularity, and much more. This is why we talk about herbal teas if wisely used, as natural remedies for all purposes that can also relax the nervous system (for example, there are some herbal teas suitable for promoting sleep) or on the contrary to give a boost of energy to the body in case of need. Therefore, herbal teas are preparations that exploit the solvent effect of hot or cold water to extract medicinal substances from plant sources of health interest.

How do they prepare?

Preparing a herbal tea is very easy! After choosing which one to do, you can prepare it in three simple steps:

1. Bring the water to a boil and then transfer it to a teacup.

2. Then add the herbs.

3. Leave to infuse for at least 5 minutes.

If necessary, filter the herbal tea and choose, according to your taste, whether to add a teaspoon of honey to sweeten. Obviously, there are small variations on the method of preparing herbal tea.

How do you keep it?

The drying of the herbs used for the herbal teas ensures that they are maintained for a long time without ever losing their properties. Despite these advantages, however, there are factors that can influence conservation: light, temperature, and shredding of herbs. Both light and temperature manage to increase the reaction of active components, while humidity also facilitates the formation of mold. On the other hand, the shredding of herbs considerably shortens the storage times, even though it is sometimes essential. Therefore, the best thing is to keep the herbs for herbal teas in jars suitable for herbal teas to be kept away from sources of light, but also of heat. Therefore, it is preferable to keep the jars away from the kitchen stove and not keep the herbs for longer than a year.

Functions

Below we will show some examples of plants that can be associated to form the basic or cardinal remedy:

- Aphrodisiac herbal teas: Ginseng, Damiana, Echinacea
- Organic herbal teas: Eucalyptus, Grindelia, Enula, Grindelia
- Cholagogue herbal tea: Dandelion, Rhubarb

- Digestive teas: lemon balm, mint
- Diuretic herbal teas: Asparagus, Horsetail
- Purifying herbal teas: fumaria , black radish, licorice , burdock
- Galactofore herbal teas: Galega, Cumin , Galega, Fennel
- Cholesterol lowering herbal teas: Ortosiphon, Matè
- Hypno-inducing herbal teas: Escolzia, Hop, Passiflora, Piscidia, Passiflora
- Hypotensive herbal teas: Mistletoe, Elderberry
- Laxative herbal teas: Senna, Buckthorn, Cascara sagrada, Rhubarb, Buckthorn
- Sedative herbal teas: Passionflower + Hawthorn.

Chapter 2: Infusion

The infusion is a liquid preparation obtained by pouring boiling water onto the vegetable source you want to extract the water-soluble component. Of all the extraction techniques, the infusion is undoubtedly the most practical and common one, thanks to the great availability of water and the simplicity of preparation. The infusion is more suitable for extracting components that degrade or are lost during boiling (e.g., essential oils); on the other hand, considering the reduced soaking times, the drug must be made up of soft and delicate fabrics (flowers and leaves), adequately chopped or reduced to powder. Once prepared, the infusion must be consumed within a short time, especially when obtained from fresh drugs. Any storage can be done in the refrigerator, without however, exceeding 24 hours.

How do you prepare it?

To prepare an infusion, you must first concentrate on the drug, which must be reduced to powder or small pieces to facilitate the intimate penetration of the solvent. Water previously brought to the boil is then poured onto the vegetable source, followed by rapid mixing and allowed to stand for a time-varying from 5 to 20 minutes depending on the drug. When preparing an infusion, it is very important to use a well-clean container, made up of inert material (generally glass or terracotta, not aluminum), and equipped with a lid (to avoid the loss of the most volatile substances). At the end of the maceration, generally protracted until the drink has cooled, the infusion is eventually filtered and promptly served. The weight/weight ratio, between the infused drug and the volume of water, normally varies from 1:25 to 1: 5 (from 4 to 20 grams for every 100 parts of water). For the preparation of a therapeutic infusion, it is very important to know the quantity of drugs, that of water, and the specific infusion time. In this sense, we can distinguish two different types of infusions: the aromatic one - characterized by an infusion time varying from 5 to 10 minutes, useful for appreciating the aromatic properties of the drug - and that of the therapeutic infusions, in which the infusion times are greater. In any case, due to the dilution of the active principles, the dosing difficulties, and the poor solubilization of some apolar substances, the infusion finds space above all in the domestic environment. At the same time, in the phytotherapy one, it is preferred in many cases to use different preparation methods or to resort directly with titrated extracts.

What are the differences between infusions and herbal teas?

Commonly these two drinks are confused; one is given the meaning of the other without ever paying attention to the differences that mainly consist of the ingredients and the preparation. Let's clarify. The herbal tea is the result of the infusion of a maximum of 6 finely chopped medicinal plants, left to infuse for 5 to 10 minutes (sometimes even up to 25 minutes, depending on the type of ingredients used) and filtered subsequently. Precisely from shredding comes the release of the active ingredients of the herbs. To be effective, the herbal tea must be composed of the main plant called cardinal remedium to add the other plants that perform the adjuvant function to the beneficial effect of the main plant. However, the infusion is the result of the infusion of flowers and leaves, therefore soft parts of the same plant. After leaving the mixture in the cup for 5-10 minutes (or up to 25 minutes as for herbal teas, it always depends on the type of plant chosen), it must be filtered carefully. For example, tea and chamomile belong to the category of infusions.

Chapter 3: Other types of preparation

Decoction

The decoction is a liquid preparation obtained by immersing a vegetable source in boiling water, to extract some active principles. In particular, the decoction is indicated for obtaining substances of herbal or pharmaceutical interest from particularly leathery drugs (bark, roots, hard leaves, seeds, etc.). However, it is not suitable for aromatic plants such as mint. It determines the evaporation of volatile oils linked to therapy, and for those rich in thermolabile active principles, which would be inactivated by heat.

To prepare a good decoction, the drug must have the appropriate dimensions and characteristics (for example, the decoction of the dried marshmallow root is made laxative by the abundant extraction of mucilage). The decoction, possibly preceded by maceration in cold water for two or three hours, is carried out by adding the parts of the plant that contain the active substances in cold water, drinkable or better still distilled, according to the prescribed quantities; bring everything to a boil and let it boil for 5-30 minutes on low heat (depending on the type of drug and needs). During this period, the herbal sources slowly release their active principles, which pass into the water together with unwanted components, some of which are then removed by filtration. Usually, one part of the drug is used every 16-20 parts of water (a ratio of 5: 100 between drug and decoction), which can be enriched with citric or hydrochloric acid in the case of alkaloid drugs. The methods of preparing the decoctions can vary significantly in relation to the source and the practitioner. For example, double decoctions can be prepared, allowing the drug to boil for a limited time, replacing the liquid and proceeding with the final decoction; in this way, in the first extract, volatile substances and those more sensitive to heat can be recovered, which would be lost with the traditional procedure. Widely used in folk medicine, decoctions do not find much space in modern herbal medicine, as prolonged boiling often leads to the inactivation of active principles or the change of their pharmacological activity.

Macerate

Macerate is a liquid preparation obtained by prolonged immersion of a vegetable source, in water or other liquids strictly at room temperature. In particular, the macerate is indicated above all for extracting active principles of herbal or pharmaceutical interest, water-soluble but thermolabile (heat-inactivated) or volatile (which are lost by evaporation). The effectiveness of maceration depends on the degree of subdivision of the drug, which must be appropriately shredded to avoid coarse cuts.

How do you prepare it?

Therefore, macerate is a rather simple extraction method, used on those medicinal plants whose active ingredients are soluble in cold water. In this regard, it is sufficient to immerse the appropriately chopped drug in the water at room temperature and then leave it to rest in a covered container, for periods ranging from a few hours to several days. The aqueous macerate is known for its ability to effectively extract mucilages from Altea's roots (protective and emollient, laxative). Arbutin from the leaves of Uva Ursina reducing - compared to the infusion - the amount of tannins extracted (which have irritant action at gastric level, while arbutin performs a urinary antiseptic activity, useful against cystitis). Before taking, the macerate must generally be carefully filtered through a strainer or a tea towel; the insoluble residue of maceration is called lees.

Compared to decoction and infusion, macerate, therefore, allows preserving heat-sensitive substances but has the disadvantage of requiring long preparation times. As a solvent for maceration, alcohol, ether, vinegar, wine, oil etc. can be used instead of water. By subjecting the drug to a whole series of subsequent macerations, an almost total recovery of its soluble components can be obtained,

Chapter 4: Herbal guide

Nature, with its innumerable remedies, offers a solution to many small health problems. The compounds contained in plants affect our body and can help us to fight anxiety and stress, find a good mood, relieve physical pain, rest better, and much more. All this, sipping a simple infusion: just knowing how to choose the right one for the problem we want to solve.

Herbs and infusions to regain energy and vitality

When we feel down, tired, and lacking in energy, or when we wake up more tired than when we went to sleep, we can find strength and vitality thanks to different plants.

Our beloved coffee is not the only stimulant that nature offers us, on the contrary. If we are experiencing a particularly stressful period, an adaptogen plant infusion can help us, while to regain the charge in a passing moment, we can opt for tonic herbs.

The main adaptogenic plants are:

- Eleutorococco
- Ginseng
- Whitania
- Schizandra

Among the herbs with tonic and stimulating action, in addition to tea and coffee we find mate and guarana.

Herbs and infusions against anxiety and bad mood

Anxiety, stress, and bad mood can manifest themselves in particular moments of our life, such as job interviews or exams, or be part of our existence for longer periods, greatly influencing our days. To calm the manifestations given by anxiety, such as palpitations, excessive sweating and a sense of fear, sedative plants come to our rescue.

Among these, in addition to the note to the common chamomile, we find:

- Hawthorn
- passionflower
- Hop
- Lavender
- Melissa
- lime

In case of bad mood, plants with a better antidepressant action are instead:

- hypericum
- Kawa kawa
- Gentian

Herbs and infusions to rest better

Resting well is necessary to face better the day and all the challenges we face every day. Unfortunately, in some periods, it can happen to struggle to fall asleep or to sleep continuously throughout the night. In these cases, it can be useful to take a Hypno-inducing infusion half an hour before going to bed to ensure a truly restful sleep. The most relaxing herbal teas and the best herbs in this case are:

- Valerian
- Hop
- Poppy
- Meliloto
- passionflower

Herbs against coughs and colds

In the case of coughs, colds, and other problems that can afflict the airways, the appropriate infusions are those with an emollient action to soothe the cough's irritations, balsamic to free the respiratory tract, antiseptic and expectorants.

The emollient infusions are prepared with:

- Altea
- Mauve
- Plantain

The best known herbs with balsamic and antiseptic action
are instead:

- Eucalyptus
- thyme
- Lavender
- Pine tree

Among the plants with expectorant action there are
instead primrose and polygala, the latter also useful for
calming the cough.

Herbs for better digestion

Digestion of food is an essential process for our body
because it allows us to assimilate the nutrients of the
foods we eat. If digestion does not take place correctly,
we can experience various symptoms, ranging from a
sense of heaviness in the stomach to abdominal swelling,
going from headache and bad mood.

Plants used in digestive infusions are:

- Roman chamomile
- Caraway
- Anise
- Fennel
- Laxative herbs

One of the most common problems among the
population of all ages is constipation. Many people suffer
from constipation due to sedentary life and poor
nutrition. When the cause of constipation can be resolved
by correcting the lifestyle, it is preferable to improve
nutrition and practice physical activity. If the stispi instead

occurs occasionally, it is possible to resort to herbs rich in mucilage that increase the fecal mass and consequently stimulate intestinal peristalsis and the evacuation of the stool. Drugs of this type are, for example, flax and psyllium seeds to be taken after infusion in water.

Herbs for menstrual cycle problems

Premenstrual syndrome and the period when menstruation occurs can cause several symptoms, including pain, irritability, swelling, and exhaustion.

The infusions that help to better cope with the premenstrual syndrome are prepared with evening primrose and cimicifuga. At the same time, in case of pain during the days of the cycle, they can be alleviated by spasmolytic drugs. These include:

- Achillea
- Roman chamomile
- Melissa
- Marjoram
- Cumin
- Herbs against cystitis

Cystitis is widespread and common inflammation of the urinary tract, especially among women. Those who have suffered or suffer from it know well what the symptoms are: a continuous urge to urinate, difficulty urinating, and suprapubic pain. In cystitis, infusions prepared with plants with antiseptic, diuretic, and spasmolytic action are used. Among these we find:

- Bearberry
- Juniper
- Bilberry and cranberry
- Weeden
- Birch
- Nettle
- Chamomile

Chapter 5: Draining drinks

1)   1) Infusion of birch and dandelion

Ingredients:
- **3 tablespoons of dried dandelion flowers**
- **2 tablespoons of dried birch leaves**
- **1 liter of water**

Put 1 liter of water in a saucepan and heat it, without ever boiling it; Add the herbs and leave to infuse for 10 minutes dried and 2 tablespoons of dried dandelion and leave for about 10 minutes.

2)   Herbs of parsley and lemon

Ingredients:
- **1 lemon**
- **1 bunch of fresh parsley**
- **1 liter of water**

put 1 liter of water in a saucepan and heat it, without ever bringing it to a boil; add the fresh parsley and leave to infuse for 10 minutes; squeeze the whole lemon and leave to rest for 30 minutes.

3) Draining anti-cellulite macerate

Ingredients:
- **Birch leaves 10 gr**
- **Pilosella leaves 10 gr**
- **Orthosyphonid leaves 10 gr**
- **Bearberry leaves 10 gr**
- **Nettle leaves 10 gr**
- **Organic honey Optional**

In a liter of water at room temperature put all the ingredients; Leave to infuse for about 6 hours so that the herbs release their nutrients and active ingredients into the water; Filter and, if you like, sweeten with a little organic honey; Drink a liter of this herbal tea throughout the day.

4) Purifying anti-cellulite herbal tea

Ingredients:
- **Orthosiphon leaves 20 gr**
- **Dandelion root 10 gr**
- **Elderflower 10 gr**
- **Artichoke leaves 10 gr**
- **Brown cane sugar Optional**

Boil 300 ml of water with all the ingredients; Leave to boil for 5 minutes and turn off the heat; When the decoction has cooled, optionally add a spoonful of brown sugar and two leaves of fresh mint; Drink 2 cups a day of this cleansing herbal tea.

5) Deflating anti-cellulite herbal tea

Ingredients:
- **Fennel seeds 15 gr**
- **Goldenrod leaves 10 gr**
- **Cherry peduncles 15 gr**
- **Nettle leaves 10 gr**
- **Organic honey Optional**

Prepare a classic hot infusion by bringing 300 ml of water to a boil; Pour the ingredients and turn off the heat, covering the saucepan with a lid; Let this infusion cool and sweeten with a spoonful of organic honey; Drink two cups of infusion at will during the day.

6) Circulated tonic anti-cellulite macerate

Ingredients:
- **Centella asiatica leaves 10 gr**
- **Butcher's broom leaves 10 gr**
- **Ivy leaves 10 gr**
- **Rosemary leaves and sprigs 10 gr**
- **Gingko biloba leaves 10 gr**
- **Organic honey Optional**

In a liter of water put 5 spoons of this preparation; Leave it to infuse for about 8 hours to allow the ingredients to release their active ingredients into the water; If you prefer, you can sweeten the herbal tea with a little organic honey; Drink two cups of this infusion per day.

7)   Draining herbal tea with cherry stalks

Ingredients:
- **1 tablespoon of chopped dried peduncles**
- **1 tea cup of water**
- **Honey (optional)**

Put the peduncles (petioles) in the cup pour over the boiling water, cover and let rest for 15 minutes. After the infusion time, filter the drink with a cloth or a colander. Sweeten to taste and enjoy between meals.

8)   Purifying herbal tea with cherry, thyme and cinnamon

Ingredients:
- **1 tbsp. Small cherry**
- **1 pinch of cinnamon powder**
- **1 teaspoon thyme**

Bring the water to the boil with the cherry stalks and let it boil on a low heat for 4 minutes. Add thyme and cinnamon, remove from the heat and leave to infuse for 5 minutes. Filter and your purifying herbal tea with cherry, thyme and cinnamon is ready! Drink in the morning.

9) Purifying herbal tea with turmeric, lemon and ginger

Ingredients:

- 1 teaspoon turmeric
- 20 g ginger (approx.)
- 1 pinch black pepper
- Coconut oil to taste (or extra virgin olive oil)
- 1/2 organic lemon

Wash the ginger root and slice it into rounds, I leave the outer skin because it is very aromatic and is sometimes used in the East in the preparation of food. Bring the water to a boil in a saucepan and add the ginger slices, simmer 3-4 minutes, i.e., make a light decoction and turn off the stove afterward. In the meantime, dissolve the teaspoon of turmeric in coconut oil (or at least extra virgin olive oil), add the pepper and a drop of hot water and add to the decoction the juice of half a lemon. Herbal tea is ready!

10) Basil herbal tea

Ingredients:

- Basil 10 leaves
- Lemons 2

Wash and dry the basil leaves. Bring the water to a boil and dip the basil and lemons cut into thin slices. Leave to brew for about 15 minutes, filter and drink throughout the day!

11) Ginger and citrus herbal tea

Ingredients:
- **1/2 ginger root**
- **Orange peel 1**
- **Grapefruit zest 1**
- **Lemon zest 1**
- **Honey 1 tsp**

Boil about 300 ml of water. Meanwhile, chop the ginger root, the orange zest, the grapefruit and the lemon. Infuse everything for at least 15 minutes, filter, add a teaspoon of honey and drink!

12) Draining infusion

Ingredients:
- **Sage 2 leaves**
- **mint 5 g**
- **Rosemary 1 sprig**
- **Chamomile flowers 1 sachet**
- **Honey 1 tbsp**

Bring a saucepan with water to the heat and add the mint, rosemary and sage, bring to a boil and cook for another 5 minutes. Turn off the heat, dip a chamomile filter and leave to infuse for 5 minutes. Filter everything and sweeten with honey. Drink hot.

13) Draining herbal tea of cherries

Ingredients:
- **20 Cherries (with relative petioles)**

Wash the cherries, remove the stalks, and set aside the stalks. Wash the cherry stones under running water. In a saucepan, add the petioles and the kernels of the cherries and add the water. Cover with the lid, bring everything to a boil and cook for 10-15 minutes. Then remove the herbal tea from the heat and, without removing the lid, let it rest for 10-15 minutes. Filter the herbal tea with cherries to remove petioles and stones.

14) Karkadè herbal tea

Ingredients:
- **1 Spoon of Karkadè**

Pour 1 tablespoon of karkade for each cup of water, pour the flowers into boiling water, turn off, cover and wait for about 10 minutes. After that, you just have to filter, leave to cool to room temperature and then put in the fridge.

15) Pineapple herbal tea

Ingredients:
- **Pineapple stem and peel**

Wash and dry the stem and peel of the pineapple carefully and then boil them in a pot of water with a lid for about twenty minutes. Then filter the infusion obtained and pour it into a bottle to drink throughout the day.

Chapter 6: Slimming drinks

1) Ginger infusion

Ingredients:

- **1 fresh rhizome of ginger**
- **1 liter of water**
- **1 slice of lemon (optional)**

Clean and chop the ginger rhizome thoroughly put 1 liter of water in a saucepan and heat it, without ever bringing it to a boil; add the chopped ginger and leave to infuse for 10-15 minutes add, if you like, a slice of lemon.

2) Mate herbal tea

Ingredients:
- **3 tablespoons of grass Mate**
- **1 liter of water**

put 1 liter of water in a saucepan and heat it, never bring it to a boil; add the mate grass and leave to infuse for 5 minutes; do not filter at the end of the infusion.

3) Slimming infusion

Ingredients:
- **Bitter orange peel 15 gr**
- **Fucus seaweed 10 gr**
- **Green tea leaves 15 gr**
- **Mallow flowers and leaves 10 gr**
- **Brown cane sugar Optional**

Prepare a classic decoction with a liter of water and 5 tablespoons of herbal tea; Let the mixture boil for 8 minutes and then let it cool completely; Sweeten with a little organic brown sugar and add some fresh mint leaves; We advise you to drink three cups a day of this preparation.

4) Green coffee herbal tea

Ingredients:
- **Green coffee beans 1**
- **teaspoon 1 cup water**

First, chop the green coffee beans in a grinder or a blender; Put the chopped grains in a cup of very hot but not boiling water, the ideal temperature would be around 80 degrees; Leave to infuse for 10 minutes, before filtering and drinking still warm.

5) Turmeric and ginger herbal tea

Ingredients:
- **Turmeric powder 1 tbsp**
- **Fresh ginger root 1 piece of about 1cm**
- **Water 250 ml**
- **Lemon juice optional**

Put 250 ml of water in a saucepan, grate the fresh ginger inside and add the turmeric powder; Boil everything for about 15 minutes before filtering and drinking; You can add a little lemon juice to the herbal tea.

6) Matè grass

Ingredients:
- **Matè grass in leaves 1 tbsp**
- **Water 1 cup**

Heat the water until it reaches a temperature of about 70 ° C; Add the herb and leave to infuse for a few minutes before filtering and drinking.

7) Mint infusion

Ingredients:
- **Fresh or dried mint leaves 1 tbsp**
- **Water 1 cup**

Boil the water, when it has reached a boil, turn off the heat and add the mint leaves; Leave the mint to infuse for about 10 minutes, being careful to cover the pan with a lid; All that remains is to filter and drink!

8)   Costume test tea

Ingredients:

- **5 g ginger (weight excluding waste)**
- **40 g pink grapefruit (weight excluding waste)**
- **2 teaspoons of green tea**

Peel the ginger, cut it into slices, and put it in a saucepan with water. Put the lid on and bring to the boil; then let it boil for about 3 minutes. Turn off the heat and wait a few minutes for the water temperature to drop. Then add the green tea leaves. Put the lid back on and leave to infuse for no more than 1 minute and a half because, otherwise, the green tea becomes very bitter. After the infusion time, add a slice of pink grapefruit without the peel and crush it to get everything out the juice. Finally, filter everything and enjoy!

9)   Honey, lemon and chilli herbal tea

Ingredients:

- **2 spicy chillies**
- **1 lemon**
- **1 tbsp honey**

Pour the water into a saucepan and bring it to a boil. In the meantime, wash the lemon under running water and cut it into slices. As soon as the water comes to a boil, pour the chilli peppers into small pieces in the pan, the slices of half a lemon and the squeezed, and filtered juice of the other half. Let it boil for about 5 minutes, then turn off the heat and filter the herbal tea with a narrow mesh

strainer. Sweeten the drink with honey and mix very well
to dissolve it. Serve the herbal tea honey lemon and hot
or cold pepper.

10) Honey herbal tea with lemon and cinnamon

Ingredients:
- **8 teaspoons honey**
- **4 teaspoons ground cinnamon**
- **16 tbsp lemon juice (squeezed and filtered)**

Pour the water into a saucepan and bring it to a boil. As
soon as it boils, pour the powdered cinnamon inside and
leave it to infuse for 10 minutes. When the herbal tea is
lukewarm, filter to eliminate the cinnamon residues and
add the squeezed and filtered lemon juice and the honey.
Stir to mix the ingredients perfectly. Serve the lemon and
cinnamon honey herbal tea and enjoy it in all its
goodness!

11) Slimming herbal tea with green tea and fennel

Ingredients:
- **1 teaspoon fennel seeds**
- **1 teaspoon green tea (leaves)**

Pour the water into a saucepan and bring it to a boil with
the lid. When it boils, add the fennel seeds and let it boil
for a couple of minutes, always with the lid so as not to
disperse the essential oils. Then turn off the heat and also
add the green tea leaves. Cover again and leave to infuse

for no more than 1 minute and a half because, otherwise, the green tea becomes very bitter. After the time of infusion, filter everything through a small dense mesh strainer and enjoy it.

12) Ginger and apple fat burning herbal tea

Ingredients:
- **Cinnamon powder 1 tsp**
- **fresh ginger root 20 g**
- **the peel of half an apple**

Pour 2 cups of water into a saucepan. Clean the ginger root and cut it into small pieces, add it to the water together with 1 teaspoon of cinnamon powder and the peel of half a red or yellow apple, as you prefer. Bring to a boil and let it boil for 3 minutes, then turn off and let the herbal tea rest for another 5 minutes. Filter the ginger, apple, and cinnamon herbal tea and drink 2 cups a day on an empty stomach then 1 in the morning just after getting up and the other in the late afternoon or the evening. Its beneficial properties will help you achieve the desired shape.

13) Fennel and cumin herbal tea

Ingredients:
- **1 teaspoon cumin seeds**
- **1 teaspoon fennel seeds**
- **1 teaspoon ground ginger**
- **1 teaspoon chamomile**
- **1 lemon zest**

Put the water in a saucepan and bring to a boil, then add the lemon zest and let it boil for 5 minutes. Add fennel, cumin, ginger and chamomile. Let it boil slowly for another 5 minutes then turn off the stove. After 20 minutes filter. Drink 2 cups a day.

14) Fat burning herbal tea

Ingredients:
- **4 cm of ginger root**
- **2 bay leaves**
- **Juice of 1 lemon**
- **10 g Turmeric powder**

Rinse the ginger, cut it into small pieces, squeeze a lemon, wash the bay leaves, and keep everything aside. Heat the water in a saucepan and bring to the boil, as soon as it boils add the ginger, bay leaf and lemon juice, boil 10 minutes, add the turmeric and let it boil for another 5 minutes, turn off the heat and leave brew another 10 minutes. Strain through a strainer. Your fat-burning herbal tea is ready to be sipped in the morning on an empty stomach, during meals, and during the day.

15) Ginseng herbal tea

Ingredients:

- **chopped ginseng root**

Put half a teaspoon of it in hot water, cover it and let it rest for ten minutes. You filter and drink. It is recommended to drink it in the morning.

Chapter 7: Purifying drinks

1) **Herbal tea with dandelion, cumin, milk thistle, mint and turmeric**

Ingredients:
- 80gr of fresh mint leaves
- 40 gr of cumin fruits
- 80 gr of turmeric powder
- 120 gr of dried dandelion leaves
- 80 gr of milk thistle
- 1 liter of water

put 1 liter of water in a saucepan and heat it, without ever bringing it to a boil; add herbs and spices, leave to infuse for 10 minutes; filter.

2) **Herbal tea with fennel**

Ingredients:
- 4 tablespoons of fennel seeds
- 1 liter of water

put 1 liter of water in a saucepan and heat it, without ever bringing it to a boil; add the fennel seeds and leave to infuse for 10-12 minutes; filter.

3) General purifying herbal tea herbal tea

Ingredients:
- **25 gr of Burdock**
- **25 gr of dandelion**
- **25 gr of Fennel**
- **25 gr of milk thistle**

Pour 250 ml of water into a saucepan, along with a spoonful of the mix of herbs; Turn on the heat, bring to the boil and boil for 5 minutes, then turn off the heat; Cover the saucepan with a lid and leave to infuse for another 10 minutes, then strain and drink.

4) Purifying herbal tea with diuretic effect
Ingredients:
- **25 gr of Artichoke (leaves)**
- **20 gr of Dandelion (root)**
- **15 gr of Malva (flowers and leaves)**
- **25 gr of Fennel (seeds)**
- **15 gr of Mint (leaves)**

Pour 250 ml of water into a saucepan, and a spoonful of the mix of herbs; Turn on the heat and boil for 3 or 4 minutes; Turn off the heat, cover the pan with a lid and leave to infuse for another 10 minutes, then strain and drink.

5) Autumn purifying and digestive decoction

Ingredients:

- **10 g Turmeric (powder)**
- **40 gr of dandelion (root)**
- **30 gr Mallow (flowers and leaves)**
- **20 gr of Sweet clover (flowering tops)**

Bring a saucepan full of water to a boil; When the water boils add 1 level spoon of the mix of plants; Wait for minutes during which the water and herbs will continue to boil together; Turn off the heat and leave to infuse for another 10 minutes; Transfer the decoction into a cup (filtering the herbs) and drink still hot.

6) Purifying decoction for the diet

Ingredients:

- **25 gr of Burdock (root)**
- **25 gr of dandelion (root)**
- **20 gr of Gramigna (rhizome)**
- **15 gr of mint (leaves)**
- **15 gr of Licorice (root)**

Boil a pot of water; When the water boils add a spoonful of the mix of plants and let it boil for 5 or 6 minutes; After 5 or 6 minutes, turn off the heat and leave to infuse for another 5 minutes; Pour the infusion into a cup (filtering the herbs) and drink it still hot.

7) Ginger and lemon infusion to cleanse the kidneys and intestines

Ingredients:

- **1 teaspoon of Bermuda grass (rhizome)**
- **1 teaspoon nettle (leaves)**
- **1 teaspoon of birch (leaves)**

Pour 200 ml of water with a teaspoon of bermuda rhizome into a saucepan, light the heat and boil for at least 3 minutes; Turn off the heat and add a teaspoon of nettle leaves and a teaspoon of birch leaves; Cover with a lid and let rest for 10 minutes, then filter and drink the herbal tea.

8) Decoction to purify the kidneys

Ingredients:

- **½ teaspoon milk thistle (seeds)**
- **½ teaspoon of dandelion (roots)**
- **½ teaspoon sage (leaves)**
- **½ teaspoon of artichoke (leaves)**

Pour 200 ml of water into a saucepan, together with half a teaspoon of milk thistle seeds and half a teaspoon a dandelion root; Turn on the heat and boil for about 5/6 minutes; Now turn off the heat, add half a teaspoon of sage leaves and half a teaspoon of artichoke leaves and cover with a lid, leaving to rest for 10 minutes; Strain and pour into a cup. Your herbal tea is ready to taste.

9)   Lemon and pineapple herbal tea

Ingredients:
- **2 lemons**
- **1 stem of pineapple**
- **pineapple peel**
- **1 spoon honey (optional)**

Peel the pineapple, remove the stem from the fruit and put it in a saucepan. Take the peel, pass it under running water then put it in the pan together with the stem. Remove the lemon peel being careful not to take the white part, and put it together with the pineapple. Add the water and bring it to a boil, lower the heat, and cook for about ten minutes. Turn off the heat and leave to steep for a couple of hours. Filter the water by removing the stem and the skins, then add the squeezed lemon juice and mix. Herbal tea is ready. Choose whether to drink it slowly throughout the day or to put it in the cup, heat it in the microwave, for example and drink it hot. You can add a spoonful of honey to make it sweeter. But this is optional.

10) Post-party infusion

Ingredients:

- **25 g Fennel seeds**
- **25 g Chamomile flowers**
- **25 g Peppermint leaves**
- **5 g Root ginger**
- **25 g Licorice root**

The water is boiled, about 150-200 ml per person, and when it has boiled, a level spoon of the mixture is introduced. The fire is turned off, everything is covered and left to infuse for about 6-8 minutes, after which it is poured and served in the cup.

11) Fennel and orange herbal tea

Ingredients:

- **50 g Fresh fennel**
- **Half organic orange peel (whole - not grated)**
- **Honey (to sweeten)**

Wash the fennel, cut it into pieces and put it in cold water in a saucepan. Put on the fire. As soon as the water boils, add the orange zest and simmer for about ten minutes. Remove from the heat, strain through a sieve and let cool before adding honey to sweeten.

12) Purifying herbal tea with laurel and anise

Ingredients:
- **2 bay leaves (fresh)**
- **2 Star anise**
- **1 teaspoon honey (optional)**

Wash the bay leaves well under running water and break them up. Pour the water into a small saucepan and add the chopped bay leaves and the two anise stars. Put the lid on and bring to the boil. Boil for 2/3 minutes (always with the lid on so as not to disperse the essential oils), then turn off the heat and leave to infuse for 5 minutes. After this time, filter everything through a dense mesh strainer. If desired, the purifying herbal tea can be sweetened with a teaspoon of honey. Serve immediately hot. Enjoy!

13) Fruit infusion

Ingredients:
- **1 Orange untreated**
- **1 Untreated apple**
- **1 cinnamon sticks**

Wash the fruit, dry it, and cut it into slices. Place it in the dryer and start it at 55 °. It will take about eight hours for the fruit to be well dried: it must be well dried to avoid risk deterioration. Let it cool and cut it into small pieces. Also, break the cinnamon. Transfer everything into an airtight jar and mix well. Leave to flavor for one week before using the preparation. Two teaspoons of preparation are used for each cup to be infused for 5 minutes in water at 95 °. If you prefer something more intense, you can add 25 grams of black Ceylon tea in leaves.

14) Nettle herbal tea

Ingredients:
- **Fresh nettle 5 leaves**
- **Honey 1 tsp**

Bring the water almost to a boil, pour it into a cup and leave to infuse the 5 nettle leaves previously washed and dried. Let it sit for about 5 - 7 minutes, after which remove the leaves and sweeten with a teaspoon of honey. Your nettle herbal tea is ready.

15) Buddhist monks herbal tea

Ingredients:
- 1 tablespoon mixture for green tea
- 1 tablespoon mixture for herbal tea based on tulsi (holy basil)
- 1 g dry ginseng root
- 10 minced mint leaves
- 1 teaspoon rosemary needles
- 1 teaspoon dried cornflower
- 1 teaspoon aloe vera juice
- 2 drops lemongrass

Take all the dry ingredients and mix them in a bowl. This dose will serve you for many doses, of course, but now we start to prepare only one. Boil a cup of water. Take a soup spoon of your herbal mix and infuse it in boiling water. Add the aloe and lemongrass. (in this case, the doses described). After the 10 minutes of infusion, remove the mix of herbs, and drink the Buddhist monks' herbal tea.

Chapter 8: Relaxing drinks

1) Mallow herbal tea

Ingredients:

- **5 teaspoons of dried flowers and mallow leaves**
- **1 liter of water**

put 1 liter of water in a saucepan and heat it, without ever bringing it to a boil; add the dried mallow and leave to infuse for 10-15 minutes; filter.

2) Relaxing goodnight infusion

Ingredients:
- **30 gr of Chamomile (flowers)**
- **20 gr of hawthorn (flowers and leaves)**
- **20 gr lemon balm (leaves)**
- **20 gr linden (flowers and leaves)**
- **10 gr of Orange Blossoms**

In a saucepan with 250 ml of boiling water, pour a spoonful of this mixture of herbs and turn off the heat; Cover this infusion and let it rest for at least 10 minutes; You can sweeten it all with a touch of organic honey.

3) Infused to promote sleep and good mood

Ingredients:

- 35 gr of Lavender (flowers)
- 35 gr lemon balm (leaves)
- 20 gr of mint (leaves)
- 10 gr of St. John's wort (flowering tops)

Bring a pot of water to the boil, turn off the heat and add a spoonful of the mix of herbs, prepared after the indicated doses; Cover this infusion and let it rest for about 8/10 minutes; Pour the infusion into a cup (filtering the herbs) and drink hot.

4) Soothing herbal tea

Ingredients:

- 4 cinnamon sticks (bark)
- 40 gr lemon balm (leaves)
- 30 gr of orange peel
- 15 gr of Chamomile (flowers)
- 15 gr of Passiflora (flowering tops)

Break a cinnamon stick and boil a piece in a saucepan full of water for 5 minutes; Turn off the heat, pour a spoonful of the mix of the remaining ingredients, cover and leave to rest for 10 minutes; Filter the herbal tea obtained and enjoy it in your favorite cup to indulge in a pampering of pure relaxation.

5) Anti-stress infusion

Ingredients:
- **30 gr of Lavender (flowers)**
- **30 gr of Passiflora (flowering tops)**
- **20 gr of Escolzia (flowers and leaves)**
- **20 gr of mint (leaves)**

Boil a pot of water; When the water boils turn off the heat, add 1 full spoonful of the mix of herbs and leave to infuse for 5/6 minutes; Pour the infusion into a cup (filtering the herbs) and drink hot.

6) Infused to sleep deeply

Ingredients:
- **25 gr of hawthorn (flowers and leaves)**
- **25 gr of Poppy (petals)**
- **25 gr of Lavender (flowers)**
- **25 gr linden (flowers and leaves)**

Boil a pot of water; When the water boils turn off the heat, add 1 full spoonful of the mix of herbs and leave to infuse for 5/6 minutes; Pour the infusion into a cup (filtering the herbs) and drink hot.

7)   Anti-stress herbal tea with saffron

Ingredients:

- Stigmas of saffron
- Honey to taste

To prepare the saffron herbal tea, boil the water. For the quantity, pour the water contained in the number of cups you want to prepare into the kettle. As soon as the water has boiled, pour it into the cups. Put a pinch of stigmas in each, crumbling your fingers a little. Leave the saffron to infuse for about ten minutes. At this point, if you want, you can filter the liquid through a narrow-mesh strainer so as to remove the saffron stigmas. I recommend tasting herbal tea with stigmas. Combine honey according to your personal taste. Mix well. The saffron anti-stress herbal tea is ready to be enjoyed: you can also drink it cold!

8) Herbal tea in the evening

Ingredients:

- linden 50 g
- Chamomile flowers 50 g
- Orange 20 g
- Hawthorn 20 g
- Poppy seeds 20 g
- verbena 10 g
- Lemon balm 10 g

Heat the water in a saucepan, and then add the herbs to the infusion for 10 minutes. Let it sit until the drink cools down to the point where you can drink it.

9) Aniseed herbal tea

Ingredients:

- 2 tablespoons anise seeds
- 1 sachet sweetener with stevia

Put some water in a saucepan. Add the anise seeds and bring to the boil. Leave to rest for 5-7 minutes. Sweeten with sweetener and consume.

10) Saffron herbal tea

Ingredients:

- Saffron in pistils (or powder) 1/2 tsp

Bring the water to a boil and pour it into a cup. Infuse the saffron for about 10 minutes. If you have used the saffron in pistils, at the end of the infusion, filter it with a narrow-mesh strainer. If you want, adjust the flavor with a spoonful of honey. Drink it hot or lukewarm so as not to disperse the beneficial effects of saffron.

11) Marjoram infusion

Ingredients:

- **dried marjoram 1 tsp**

In a saucepan, bring the water to a boil, turn off the gas, add the marjoram, turn well and leave to infuse for 10 minutes, filter the infusion and drink.

12) Cinnamon and mandarin herbal tea

Ingredients:

- **1 sachet of black tea**
- **1 Mandarin**
- **1 teaspoon ground cinnamon**

Peel the tangerine by removing the outer peel and divide into wedges. Boil the mandarin with the cinnamon for a couple of minutes, then pour the liquid into a bowl by filtering it. Infuse the tea for at least 3 minutes and sweeten to taste.

13) Relaxing herbal tea

Ingredients:

- **1 teaspoon chamomile flowers (dried)**
- **1 teaspoon Melissa**
- **½ teaspoons Lavender**

Put the water in a saucepan and bring it to a boil. Prepare the herbs and pour boiling water over them; cover with a lid to avoid dispersing the essential oils and leave to infuse for 10 minutes. After the infusion time, filter the whole with a small dense mesh strainer. Sweeten the relaxing herbal tea with a teaspoon of honey (or with brown sugar) and drink it hot or at room temperature.

14) Chamomile and parsley herbal tea

Ingredients:
- **A sprig of parsley (Chopped)**
- **A sachet of chamomile tea**

Boil the water and add both the sachet of chamomile and the parsley, better if chopped and then leave it to infuse for at least ten minutes.

15) Hop tea, lavender and escolzia

Ingredients:
- **a teaspoon of flowering hop tops**
- **1 of dried lavender bud**
- **1 bud of escolzia**

Boil the water, turn off, pour the herbs and leave to stand covered for 5 minutes. Filter and drink.

16) Melissa and Valerian herbal tea

Ingredients:
- **2 teaspoons of lemon balm**
- **2 of valerian**

Boil the water, turn off, pour the herbs and leave to stand covered for 5 minutes. Filter and drink.

Chapter 9: Energy Drinks

1) Lemongrass herbal tea

Ingredients:
- **3 tablespoons of dried lemongrass**
- **a few mint leaves**
- **1 liter of water**

put 1 liter of water in a saucepan and heat it, without ever bringing it to a boil; add the dried lemongrass and leave to infuse for 10 minutes; filter and add, if desired, the mint leaves.

2) Rosemary herbal tea

Ingredients:
- **2 sprigs Rosemary**
- **1 teaspoon honey**

To prepare the herbal tea with rosemary, simmer the rosemary in hot water for 10 minutes, after washing it thoroughly under cold running water. Filter it, let it rest for two minutes covered, sweeten with honey. Your natural remedy is ready to be consumed.

3)   Fresh Mint Infusion with Lemon Juice

Ingredients:
- **6 leaves Fresh mint**
- **2 slices organic lemon**
- **2 tablespoons lemon juice**
- **q.s. Sugar cane**

Pour the water into a pot and bring to the boil. In the meantime wash the mint leaves and the organic lemon. Cut two central slices of the lemon. Squeeze half. When the water boils, turn off the heat and add the mint leaves, the juice and the slices of lemon. Cover and let rest 10/15 minutes. Leave to cool and if you like, sugar to taste.

4)   Ginkgo biloba herbal tea

Ingredients:
- **40g of ginkgo biloba leaves,**
- **30g of rosemary,**
- **30g of eleutherococcus root**

Place the water to boil in a saucepan. Pour the ingredients, and leave to infuse for 10 minutes, filter. Drink twice a day after main meals.

5) Orange herbal tea

Ingredients:
- **5 tablespoons of star anise**
- **2 tablespoons of juniper berries**
- **2 tablespoons of sweet orange peel**
- **a spoonful of licorice root**

Pour all the ingredients into cold water and bring to a boil. Turn off to leave to infuse for one minute. Filter, drink.

6) Decoction with greater burdock, artichoke, licorice and dandelion

Ingredients:
- **A teaspoon of greater burdock**
- **A teaspoon of dried artichoke leaves**
- **A teaspoon of licorice**
- **A teaspoon of dandelion**

Boil the water, then add the herbs indicated except the licorice, and boil for 5 minutes. Turn off the heat, add the licorice, cover and leave to infuse for 5 minutes. Filter the preparation, and drink a cup in the morning and one after lunch.

7)   Rosehip infusion

Ingredients:
- **Dried rosehip berries**

Chop the berries and boil the water. Pour the water into a cup and add a spoonful of berries, leaving to infuse for about 10 minutes. Strain, add a little honey and consume two cups a day.

8)   Peppermint, rose and tea infusion

Ingredients:
- **3 peppermint leaves**
- **3 rose petals**
- **2 pinches of green tea**

Heat the water in a saucepan, and before boiling, pour it into a previously heated teapot in which mint leaves, rose petals and tea are already found. Cover the teapot and leave to infuse for about 5 minutes. Pour the filtered herbal tea into a cup. Drink in the morning

9)   Forest fruit tea

Ingredients:
- **15g of blueberry**
- **15 g of black currant**
- **10 g of hibiscus**
- **10 g of elderberries**
- **10 g peppermint**

Mix the dried ingredients and use 2 teaspoons in a cup of boiling water. Leave to infuse for 5 minutes and drink.

**10) Energetic herbal tea with green tea and
grapefruit**

Ingredients:

- **2 teaspoons of green tea leaves**
- **1 grapefruit zest**
- **1 slice of fresh ginger**

Boil all the ingredients in a saucepan for 5 minutes.
Consumed after main meals, it speeds up the metabolism
by promoting the transformation of fats into energy.

11) Coriander and manna herbal tea

Ingredients:

- **1 tablespoon of coriander seeds**
- **1 sachet of manna powder**

Simmer the water in a saucepan with coriander seeds for
5 minutes, then strain and let it cool. At this point,
dissolve a sachet of manna powder in the herbal tea. Stir
and drink in the morning.

12) Coffee infusion

Ingredients:
- **a cup of coffee**
- **a pinch of ginger**
- **a pinch of cinnamon**
- **a pinch of sweet paprika**
- **a spoonful of honey**

Add all the ingredients to the boiling coffee, mix, cover and leave to infuse for 10 minutes. Without filtering drink the infusion in the middle of the morning.

13) Eleutherococcus herbal tea

Ingredients:
- **Eleutherococcus Root 30gr**
- **Mint 10gr**
- **Fenugreek 30gr**
- **Maca 30gr**

Boil a pot of water; When the water boils add 1 full spoonful of the mix of herbs and roots, then let it boil for 2 minutes; Turn off the heat and leave to infuse for another 10 minutes; Transfer the infusion into a cup (filtering the herbs) and drink.

Chapter 10: Digestive drinks

1) Digestive and deflating infusion

Ingredients:
- **25 gr of Caraway (seeds)**
- **25 gr of green anise (seeds)**
- **15 gr of Chamomile (flowers)**
- **25 gr of Fennel (seeds)**
- **10 gr Mallow (flowers and leaves)**

Heat 250/300 ml of water in a saucepan and bring it to a boil; Turn off the heat and transfer the water to a cup or, if you have one, to an herbal tea that can maintain the heat of the herbal tea during the infusion; Pour a spoonful of the herb mix and leave to infuse for 10 minutes; Strain and drink the hot herbal tea. You can sweeten it with a little honey if you wish.

2)   Aromatic digestive decoction

Ingredients:
- 10 gr of bitter orange (zest)
- 15 gr of star anise (seeds)
- 15 gr of mint (leaves)
- 10 gr of chopped flax seeds
- 20 gr of Fennel (seeds)
- 10 gr of Sage (leaves)
- 20 gr of Liquorice (root)

Boil a pot of water; When the water boils, pour a spoonful of the mix of ingredients and leave to boil for 5 minutes; After 5 minutes, turn off the heat and leave to brew for about 10 minutes; Pour into a cup (filtering the herbs) and drink still hot.

3)   Against acidity infusion

Ingredients:
- 30 gr of mint (leaves)
- 40 gr of Fennel (seeds)
- 10 gr Mallow (flowers and leaves)
- 20 gr of Liquorice (root)

Bring 250 ml of water to the boil; When the water boils add 1 tablespoon of the herb mix and let it boil for 2 or 3 minutes, then turn off the heat; Leave the plants to infuse for 10 minutes; Finally, pour the infusion into a cup by filtering it.

4) Digestive and deflating decoction with fennel

Ingredients:
- 10 gr lemon balm (leaves)
- 50 gr of Fennel (seeds)
- 20 gr of Psyllium (seeds)
- 20 gr of green anise (seeds)

Boil a pot of water and add 1 full spoonful of the mix of herbs, let it boil for at least 2 or 3 minutes; Turn off the heat and keep the herbal mix infused for another 10 minutes; Pour the infusion into a cup, filter the herbs and drink still hot. If you like it, you can prepare 1 liter of it to drink during the day. In this case, take 20 grams of the mix of herbs in 1 liter of water and proceed as described above.

5) Digestive and warming herbal tea

Ingredients:
- 1 cm of fresh ginger (root)
- 1 piece of orange (zest)
- 1 cm of Cinnamon (stick)
- 1 star anise berry

Pour 250/300 ml of water into a saucepan and bring it to the first boil; At this point add the cinnamon, the star anise and the ginger root deprived of the outer skin; Let it simmer for about ten minutes, then turn off the heat and filter; Add the orange zest and sip the still hot herbal tea.

6)   Fennel and coriander decoction

Ingredients:
- **Fennel seeds 25 g**
- **Coriander seeds 15 gr**
- **Mallow flowers and leaves 10 gr**

Bring 300 ml of water to a boil in a saucepan; Pour in all the ingredients and leave to infuse for at least 5 minutes; Strain through a strainer and drink after the main meals.

7)   Deflating herbal tea with anise, artichoke and lemon

Ingredients:
- **Anise seeds 25 g**
- **Star anise 10 gr**
- **Artichoke leaves 15 gr**
- **Lemon 1 zest**

Take the healing herbs and mix them to obtain a homoegenic compound; At this point, prepare a saucepan with about 250 g of boiling water and pour a spoonful of this deflating herbal tea and a slice of lemon; Leave to infuse for 7 minutes, filter and drink after the main meals; You can sweeten everything with a teaspoon of honey.

8)   Mint, dandelion and birch herbal tea

Ingredients:
- **Mint leaves 15 g**
- **Dandelion leaves 15 gr**
- **Dandelion root 10 gr**
- **Birch leaves 10 gr**

To make this deflating herbal tea, take a saucepan and bring the herbal mixture of this herbal tea to a boil; Leave to boil for 2 or 3 minutes and then turn off the heat; Cover the saucepan with a lid and leave to infuse 5-6 minutes; Strain through a strainer and sweeten with a generous teaspoon of organic raw cane sugar.

9)   Deflating herbal tea with cumin, licorice and mallow

Ingredients:
- **Cumin seeds 20 g**
- **Licorice root 20 gr**
- **Mallow flowers 10 gr**

After having combined cumin, licorice and mallow in a glass jar, mix these herbs with a wooden spoon to obtain a homogeneous mixture; Take a saucepan and put on the fire about 250 ml of water; Once brought to the boil, pour a spoonful full of this deflating herbal tea and turn off the heat; cover with a lid and leave to infuse for 7-8 minutes; Filter and sweeten with honey or organic brown sugar.

10) Herbal tea with ginger, lemon balm and verbena

Ingredients:
- **Lemon balm leaves 15 g**
- **Verbena leaves 15 gr**
- **Ginger 5 gr**
- **Fennel seeds 15 gr**

After mixing the lemon balm, the verbena and the fennel in a glass jar put on the fire about 300 ml of water and bring it to the boil; At this point, pour a spoonful of herbal tea and a slice of fresh ginger; leave to boil for a few minutes and then turn off the heat; leave to infuse for about 10 minutes and filter. Your deflating herbal tea is ready! You can drink this infusion after meals and during the day, up to 4 cups.

11) Lemon and celery herbal tea

Ingredients:
- **2 celery stalks**
- **1 lemon**

Pour the water into a saucepan and bring it to a boil. As soon as the water boils, dive into the celery sticks and leave them to infuse for about 10 minutes. After this time, turn off the heat and let the herbal tea cool down. After about 30 minutes, filter it and add the squeezed and filtered lemon juice. Mix everything well to mix the ingredients, then drink the lemon and celery herbal tea, or, if you prefer, you can sweeten it.

12) Digestive herbal tea to deflate after meal

Ingredients:
- 1 tuft of fresh fennel or fennel seeds
- 1 teaspoon ground cinnamon
- 1 organic lemon
- 4 teaspoons honey

For the digestive herbal tea to deflate after a meal, we take the water and put it in a saucepan. We combine the zest of half a lemon, the fresh fennel,or in seeds and the cinnamon. We boil for 5 minutes, then turn off and leave for 20 minutes. We filter the herbal tea and add the honey, then stir until it dissolves completely. We serve the herbal tea in cups accompanied by a slice of lemon. Let's serve it and taste it.

13) Sage and Lemon Digestive Herbal Tea

Ingredients:
- 1 organic lemon
- 8 sage leaves
- 1 teaspoon ground ginger
- 1 tablespoon Acacia honey

Let's take the water and put it in a pot. We add the sage and the zest of the lemon, trying to avoid the white part of the zest; otherwise, the herbal tea will be bitter. Bring to the boil for 10 minutes, also adding the powdered ginger. Once the herbal tea is ready, let's filter it, add the honey, and dissolve. Add the lemon juice and mix. Let the herbal tea cool down and serve it. We can double the quantity of ingredients, and then put it in a bottle, keep it in the fridge and use it if necessary. You can also drink it cold.

14) Post binge macerate

Ingredients:
- **1/2 teaspoon bicarbonate**
- **20 ml Lemon juice**

Pour the water into a glass, add the lemon juice and baking soda. Turn vigorously with the spoon and drink immediately, with all the foam.

15) Digestive herbal tea with cinnamon and star anise

Ingredients:
- **3 star anise berries**
- **1 cinnamon sticks (4-5cm)**
- **2 teaspoons wildflower honey**

Pour the water into a saucepan, add the vanilla pod, and the star anise. Cover with the lid and bring to a boil over medium heat. As soon as it reaches boiling point, turn off the heat and leave to infuse for 10 minutes. After the infusion time, filter the herbal tea with a narrow mesh strainer directly into the cups. Add one teaspoon per cup of honey to sweeten and turn with the teaspoon to dissolve completely. Sip the still hot digestive herbal tea cinnamon and star anise.

Chapter 11: Drinks that help lower cholesterol

1)   Herbal tea to lower cholesterol

Ingredients:
- **Dandelion (root) ½ tsp**
- **Burdock (root) ½ tsp**
- **Artichoke (leaves) 1 tsp**
- **Milk thistle (seeds) ½ tsp**
- **Chicory (leaves) ½ tsp**

First put 200 ml of water in a saucepan together with the dandelion root, the burdock root and the milk thistle seeds; Turn on the heat and boil for about 5 minutes on low heat; After five minutes, turn off the heat ,and add the artichoke and chicory leaves; Cover and leave to infuse for 10 minutes, then filter and drink. Given the bitter taste of the drink, if you like it, you can sweeten it with a teaspoon of honey.

2)   Artichoke herbal tea

Ingredients:
- **70 g Artichokes**
- **2 teaspoons honey**
- **to taste lemon juice**

To prepare the artichoke herbal tea, boil the water in a saucepan and add the artichoke leaves and also the stems cut into small pieces if you have them. Leave to boil for 15 minutes, then turn off the heat and leave to infuse for 5

minutes. Filter the artichoke herbal tea, add the honey
and lemon juice.

3) Citrus herbal tea with ginger and cinnamon

Ingredients:
- **Fresh ginger 6 pieces**
- **Half orange peel**
- **Zest of 1 lemon**
- **Cinnamon powder (o) 1 pinch**
- **Water 700 ml**
- **Honey or other sweetener (optional) to taste**
- **Juice of 1 lemon**
- **Half orange juice**

To prepare the herbal tea, start cutting the orange zest,
being careful not to take the white, which could make our
drink bitter. Repeat the same operation with the lemon.
In a saucepan, boil the water with the slices of ginger, add
the orange and lemon zest, and add a cinnamon pinch. If
you want, you can also use the cinnamon in the berry,
just a small piece. Cover the saucepan with the lid and let
it boil for 5 minutes. Add the citrus juice, then when
cooked, turn off the heat and let stand for 15 minutes.
Filter the herbal tea and serve it, accompanied by a few
slices of orange and lemons on the edge of the cup. If you
prefer a slightly sweeter flavor, you can add a little honey,
brown sugar, or other sweeteners

4)   Ginger herbal tea with lime and apple

Ingredients:
- **Peel of an organic apple**
- **1 Lime**
- **50 g Fresh ginger**
- **1 tsp honey**

Bring the water to a boil in a saucepan, add the cut ginger, the peel of an organic apple and the squeezed lime. Continue cooking for a few minutes. Turn off and add the honey. Consume the herbal tea with lime ginger and warm apple.

5)   Herbal tea with canary seed

Ingredients:
- **Canary seed 15g**

Boil water and canary seeds in a saucepan. They have to boil together for 10 minutes. It must then be sweetened and drunk without filtering. You should drink this herbal tea before going to bed or on an empty stomach.

6)   Amaranth infusion

Ingredients:
- **1 handful of tender amaranth leaves**

Let both ingredients boil for 5 minutes. Turn off the heat and cover with a lid, leaving the infusion to rest for at least 5 minutes. Strain and drink mid-morning. Repeat mid-afternoon.

7)   Dandelion herbal tea

Ingredients:

- **1 punch of dandelion**

As with any other infusion, we boil the water with the herb and let it cool before filtering, then sweetening and drinking.

8)   Tamarind herbal tea

Ingredients:

- **1 tamarind**
- **A few drops of lemon**

Peel the tamarind and cut it into pieces. Boil the pulp with water for at least 15 minutes. Add the lemon and drink including the pieces of fruit. It is recommended to take one cup on an empty stomach and another before going to sleep.

9)   Garlic herbal tea

Ingredients:

- **2 cloves of garlic**
- **1 green tea bag**
- **The juice of half a lemon**

Chop the raw garlic and put it in the water with the tea bag. Let stand for 5 minutes, strain and add the lemon juice. Drink the infusion once on an empty stomach and another before going to sleep.

Chapter 12: Drinks against cystitis

1) Mallow and bearberry herbal tea

Ingredients:
- **Mallow flowers and leaves 1 tbsp**
- **Bearberry 1 tbsp**

Boil 200 ml of water in a saucepan; Turn off the heat and pour a spoonful of leaves and flowers of mallow and a spoonful of bearberry leaves; Cover with a lid and let stand for 10 minutes, then strain and drink.

2) Blueberry and chamomile herbal tea

Ingredients:
- **Chamomile flower heads 1 tbsp**
- **Cranberry leaves 1 tbsp**

Pour 200 ml of water into a saucepan and bring to the boil; Turn off the heat and pour the chamomile flower heads and the cranberry leaves; Cover and let stand for 10 minutes, then strain and drink.

3) Corn and mint herbal tea

Ingredients:
- **Stigmas of corn 1 tbsp**
- **Mint leaves 1 tbsp**

Pour 200 ml of water and a spoonful of corn stigmas into a saucepan; Turn on the heat and boil for 10 minutes from boiling; Turn off the heat and add the spoonful of mint leaves; Cover with a lid and let stand for 10 minutes before filtering and drinking.

4) Bearberry tea

Ingredients:
- **30gr Corn stigmas**
- **30gr Bearberry (leaves)**
- **10gr Mint**
- **30gr Horsetail**

Mix the herbs in a bowl. Boil a small pot of water. Add 1 tablespoon of mixed herbs and boil for 3 minutes. Turn off the heat and leave to infuse for 15 minutes in a covered saucepan. Pour the filtered infusion into a cup.

5) Mallow and marigold soothing herbal tea

Ingredients:
- **20 grams of dried mallow**
- **10 grams of calendula**

Bring a liter of water to a boil, leave the two herbs to infuse for about 7 minutes; filter and drink up to three times during the day. The ideal is to keep it warm in a thermal jug.

6) Cranberry herbal tea

Ingredients:

- **About 20 grams of dried cranberry fruits**

Bring 200 ml of water to the boil, enough for a normal-sized cup; add a teaspoon of dried cranberries; leave to infuse for about 10 minutes, then filter and drink hot; up to three cups a day between meals are indicated.

7) Echinacea decoction

Ingredients:

- **1 tablespoon of echinacea roots**

Pour the chopped root into cold water, light the fire and bring 200 ml or a cup of water to the boil. Boil a few minutes and turn off the heat. Cover and leave to infuse for about 10 minutes, filter and drink.

8) Decoction with Malva, Erica and Meadowsweet

Ingredients:

- **20 gr of wild mallow leaves and flowers**
- **10 gr of heather leaves**
- **10 gr of flowering meadowsweet tops**

Prepare the decoction by boiling the herbs in the water for 5-10 minutes. Leave to rest for about ten minutes, then filter. Take 2-3 cups a day between meals.

9)   Frangula herbal tea

Ingredients:
- **Bark frangula 40 g**
- **Flax seeds 40 g**
- **Star anise 10 gr**
- **Licorice 10 g**

Bring the water to the boil with the herbal mixture and leave to infuse for ten minutes. Strain and drink lukewarm.

Chapter 13: Laxative drinks

1) **Mallow, lemon balm and coriander laxative infusion**

Ingredients:
- **Mallow flowers and leaves 20 g**
- **Coriander seeds 15 gr**
- **Lemon balm leaves 15 gr**

Bring 300 ml of water to a boil in a saucepan; Pour a tablespoon of herbal tea with mallow, lemon balm and coriander and leave to infuse for 7-8 minutes; Drink up to 3 cups a day after meals, also to perform an effective purifying action on the body. You can sweeten the herbal tea with a little honey.

2) **Flaxseed, licorice and fennel based decoction**

Ingredients:
- **Flax seeds 25 g**
- **Fennel seeds 20 gr**
- **Licorice root 5 gr**

Take a saucepan with 300 ml of water and bring them to a boil; Then pour a spoonful of the flaxseed, fennel, and licorice root mixture; Leave to infuse until the water has cooled. In this way, you will allow time for flax seeds to release the mucilages useful for promoting intestinal transit; At this point, strain and drink two cups a day.

3) Laxative herbal tea with psyllium, dandelion and artichoke seeds

Ingredients:
- **Psyllium seeds 20 g**
- **Artichoke leaves 5 gr**
- **Dandelion root 15 gr**
- **Mint leaves 10 gr**

After mixing all the ingredients , bring 250 ml of water to the boil; Turn off the heat and pour a spoonful of herbal tea with psyllium, dandelion, and artichoke; Leave to infuse until the water has cooled, then filter. You can sweeten the herbal tea with a spoonful of honey or brown cane sugar; Drink two cups a day and at least a liter of water to activate the properties of the herbal tea.

4) Rhubarb, fennel and mint laxative herbal tea

Ingredients:
- **Rhubarb root 15 g**
- **Fennel root 15 gr**
- **Mint leaves 10 gr**
- **Mallow flowers and leaves 10 gr**

After mixing rhubarb, fennel, mint and mallow in a glass jar, put on the fire about 300 ml of water and bring it to the boil; At this point, pour a spoonful of herbal tea and leave to infuse for 5 minutes; Drink a cup in the evening before bedtime; You can sweeten the herbal tea with a little organic brown sugar.

5) Senna, mint and cumin macerated

Ingredients:
- 2 grams of senna leaves
- 150 ml of hot water
- a few mint leaves
- some cumin seeds

The senna leaves are left to macerate in hot, but not boiling, water, adding mint leaves and cumin seeds for about an hour. It is filtered and drunk in the evening or in the morning.

6) Composite infusion to regulate the intestine

Ingredients:
- a teaspoon of mallow
- a teaspoon of chamomile flowers
- a pinch of fennel seeds
- half a teaspoon of buckthorn
- half a teaspoon of licorice
- some anise seeds

Mix the ingredients together, bring a pot of water to the boil, leave it to rest for about 10 minutes, filter and consume in the evening before bedtime. An excellent composite herbal tea, which gives great relief to the intestinal mucosa.

Chapter 14: Anti-inflammatory drinks

1)   Ginger and lemon herbal tea

Ingredients:
- **1 cm of ginger root**
- **½ lemon (the juice)**
- **2 teaspoons honey (preferably acacia)**

Peel the ginger and cut it into slices. Put it in a saucepan with water and simmer for about 5 minutes. Turn off the heat, add the lemon juice and stir. Filter the ginger herbal tea and pour it into the cups. Add 1 teaspoon of honey per cup, mix and serve.

2)   Elderflower infusion

Ingredients:
- **2 tsp elderberry flowers**

Put to heat the water and once it is hot insert your sachet and leave for 5 minutes. Drink when it is still hot.
Excellent for those who are influenced. Your herbal tea is ready.

3)   Orange and cinnamon honey decoction

Ingredients:
- **Honey 30g**
- **2 Organic oranges**
- **1 cinnamon sticks**
- **2 Star anise**
- **Cloves 1**
- **Lemon juice to taste**

Put 500 ml of water in a saucepan. A well-washed organic orange in thin slices. The juice of 1 lemon and the juice of 1 orange. Add a cinnamon stick, star anise, and cloves. Allow 5 minutes for the boil to start, then turn off and rest for 5 minutes. With these doses, you get 2/3 cups of hot orange and herbal honey teas.

4)   Herbal tea cinnamon ginger and cloves

Ingredients:
- **1 fresh ginger (more or less 3 cm)**
- **6 Cloves**
- **1 cinnamon sticks**
- **2 teaspoons honey**

To prepare the herbal tea, cinnamon, ginger, and cloves, first, boil the water in a saucepan. In the meantime, peel the ginger root and cut approximately 3 cm into thin slices, set aside. Chop the cinnamon stick, and once the water has boiled, add the cinnamon, ginger, and cloves to the inside. Leave to boil for 3 or 4 minutes, then turn off the heat and leave to infuse, covering with a lid to prevent the aromas from dispersing. After 10 minutes, filter the cinnamon, ginger, and clove herbal tea and sweeten with honey. You can serve it freshly-prepared hot or leave it at room temperature.

5)   Marigold and lemon balm macerate

Ingredients:
- **2 tablespoons of calendula flowers**
- **10 lemon balm leaves**
- **1 lime**

To prepare the calendula and lemon balm infusion, bring 2 liters of water to the boil. Dip the marigold flowers and put out the fire. Leave to infuse for 10 minutes. Filter the drink and pour it into a glass bottle. Leave to cool to room temperature. Add the well-washed and dried lemon balm leaves, and add the sliced lime. Transfer to the fridge and serve cold.

6)   Infusion of garlic and lemon

Ingredients:
- **1 garlic**
- **1 lemon**

Wash the lemon, preferably with a thick peel, and put it whole in a small saucepan, so that the amount of water can cover it. Then, add the garlic clove. Bring to a boil and let it boil for 7 minutes, no more. Do not raise the flame too much, and do not extend the boiling time. Remove the saucepan from the heat, remove the lemon and the clove of garlic and let it cool.

7)   Infusion of olive leaves

Ingredients:
- **Dried olive leaves 5 g**

Boil the leaves in water for a few minutes, let stand and cool, then filter and drink. The generally recommended dose is one cup per day.

8)   Sage infusion

Ingredients:
- **5 leaves dried sage**
- **Lemon juice A few drops**
- **Honey (optional) 1 tsp**

Bring the water to a boil and leave the dried sage leaves to infuse for about 10 minutes, filter and add a few drops of lemon juice and, if you wish, a teaspoon of honey. Let it cool down and drink.

9)   Herbal tea with fennel seeds

Ingredients:
- **1 teaspoon fennel seeds**

Bring a pan containing 200 ml of water to a boil, then leave the seeds to infuse for about 15 minutes with a lid.

10) Herbal tea of dried figs and honey

Ingredients:
- **200 g Dried figs**
- **Honey (acacia, sunflower**

Take a saucepan with high sides and pour 1 liter of natural water inside. Cut the figs in half lengthwise and put them in the water. Cover the saucepan with a lid and put it on the fire, bringing the water to a boil. When the water boils, lower the flame to the minimum and cook for about 40 minutes. At the end of the indicated time, the dried fig water is ready to be drunk, adding 1 - 2 teaspoons of honey to each cup you drink.

11) Ginger and turmeric herbal tea

Ingredients:
- **Fresh ginger (a piece)**
- **Fresh turmeric (a piece)**
- **Black pepper (some grains)**
- **3 tsp honey**
- **2 slices Lemon**

Put the water to heat, but without letting it boil. In the meantime, cut a piece of ginger (about 1 cm), peel it and slice it. Also, cut the turmeric (about 2 cm), peel it and cut it into small pieces. When the water is hot (but not boiling), add the ginger, turmeric, black peppercorns, and leave to infuse for at least 10 minutes. (Obviously the longer the infusion time, the more concentrated and strong the flavor will be). Sweeten with honey. Add the lemon slices and get ready to sip your ginger and turmeric herbal tea.

12) Herbal tea with fennel, bay leaf and lemon

Ingredients:
- **20 gr of fennel seeds**
- **The juice of one lemon**
- **3 bay leaves**

In a saucepan, bring the water to the boil in which you will have put the fennel seeds and the bay leaf. Boil for 15 minutes. After the time, add the lemon juice, filter the herbal tea by transferring it to a cup and sweeten it, if you prefer, with 1 or 2 teaspoons of honey.

13) Apple and cinnamon herbal tea

Ingredients;
- **1 red apple (peel only)**
- **2/3 cm Cinnamon sticks**
- **3 Cloves**

In a saucepan, put the water and bring it to a boil. When it boils, add the apple peel, the cinnamon stick, and the cloves. Boil for 5 minutes with the lid on so as not to disperse the essential oils. After this time, turn off the heat and leave to infuse for another 10 minutes. Filter everything through a small dense mesh strainer. The apple and cinnamon herbal tea are ready to be enjoyed.

14) Infusion of rose petals

Ingredients:
- **Dried Rose Petals 1 tbsp**

Take the rose petals and put them in a bowl with cold water, but only for a few moments. Dry them with kitchen paper. Put the petals in a teacup, cover them with boiling water, cover it, and leave to infuse for about 10 minutes. Filter everything and, if you want, sweeten with a teaspoon of honey. Drink the herbal tea of warm rose petals.

15) Apple and lemon herbal tea

Ingredients:
- **1/2 Royal Gala apples**
- **1/2 Lemons**

Wash the apple thoroughly, remove the core and cut it into slices. Boil the water needed for two cups of herbal tea, turn off and add the sliced apple and leave to infuse for about 4 minutes, add the lemon juice and pour the herbal tea into the cup.

Conclusion

With the lowering of temperatures it also brings some advantages, among them the possibility of tasting infusions, herbal teas that not only help us to fight the cold and take a sweet moment for ourselves, but they can support our body thanks to their beneficial properties. Precisely for this reason it is important to understand what the characteristics of these drinks are and the best way to enhance them using the right method. Nature, with its innumerable remedies, offers a solution to many small health problems. All this, while sipping a simple infusion or herbal tea, just know how to choose the right one for the problem we want to solve. Furthermore, in this guide, you have also discovered some recipes of cold infusions to taste during the summer. Integrate infusions and herbal teas into your life and find out how they can be useful for your well-being.